KID-FRIENDLY BRAINY FOODS

120 nutritious delights to fuel growing minds

ELLIE HOUSTON

Copyright © 2023 by Ellie Houston

All rights reserved.
No part of this book may be reproduced, stored in a retrieval system, or transmitted in any form or by any means, electronic, mechanical, photocopying, recording, scanning, or otherwise, without the prior written permission of the author, except for brief quotations in critical reviews or articles.

TABLE OF CONTENT

INTRODUCTION

In the whirlwind of parenting, there is a common thread that unites us all: the deep desire to provide our children with the very best, especially when it comes to their health and development. As parents, we're champions of growth, guardians of well-being, and stewards of vibrant young minds.

The cornerstone of this noble endeavour is the food we serve our children. It's the foundation upon which they build their physical strength, emotional resilience, and, crucially, cognitive prowess. In *Kid-Friendly Brainy Foods*, we embark on a culinary journey that places the spotlight on the vital role of nutritious food for growing minds. We delve into the science behind brain-boosting ingredients and explore the essential nutrients that fuel cognitive function.

Our mission is clear: to empower parents, caregivers, and educators with the knowledge to nourish young minds effectively. We aim to provide a treasure trove of kid-friendly recipes designed not only to delight their taste buds but also to optimize their brainpower. With this eBook, you'll discover that preparing brain-boosting meals can be both enjoyable and rewarding.

HEALTHY KID-FRIENDLY BRAINY RECIPES

1. Brain-Boosting Breakfast Parfait

Ingredients:

Greek yogurt

Mixed berries (strawberries, blueberries, raspberries)

Honey

Granola

Preparation:

In a glass or jar, layer Greek yogurt, mixed berries, and a drizzle of honey.

Top with granola for added crunch.

2. Veggie-Packed Egg Muffins

Ingredients:

Eggs

Chopped spinach

Diced bell peppers

Diced tomatoes

Shredded cheese

Salt and pepper

Preparation:

Whisk eggs in a bowl and season with salt and pepper.

Grease a muffin tin and distribute chopped vegetables evenly.

Pour the egg mixture over the vegetables.

Top with shredded cheese.

Bake for 15 to 20 minutes, or until set, at 350°F/175°C.

3. Nutty Banana Brain Pancakes

Ingredients:

Pancake mix (whole-grain if possible)

Mashed bananas

Chopped nuts (e.g., walnuts, almonds)

Maple syrup

Preparation:

Prepare pancake batter according to package instructions.

Stir in mashed bananas and chopped nuts.

Cook pancakes on a griddle.

Drizzle with maple syrup.

4. Brainy Veggie Quesadillas

Ingredients:

Whole-wheat tortillas

Shredded cheese

Sliced bell peppers

Sliced zucchini

 Sliced tomatoes

Salsa

Preparation:

Place a tortilla in a heated skillet.

Sprinkle with cheese and add sliced vegetables.

Top with another tortilla.

Cook until tortillas are golden brown and cheese is melted.Serve with salsa.

5. Brain-Boosting Blueberry Muffins

Ingredients:

Whole-wheat flour

Baking powder

Baking soda

Ground flaxseed

Blueberries

Greek yogurt

Honey

Preparation:

In a bowl, mix whole-wheat flour, baking powder, baking soda, and ground flaxseed.

Stir in blueberries.

Combine honey and Greek yogurt in a separate bowl. Combine wet and dry ingredients.

Spoon into muffin cups and bake at 350°F (175°C) for 15-20 minutes.

6. Superfood Peanut Butter and Banana Sandwich

Ingredients:

Whole-grain bread

Peanut butter (or almond butter)

Sliced bananas

Chia seeds

Honey

Preparation:

Take a piece of wholegrain bread and spread it with peanut butter.

Add some chia seeds, sliced bananas, and honey drizzle on top.

To make a sandwich, place another slice of bread on top.

7. Brainy Turkey and Veggie Roll-Ups

Ingredients:

Sliced turkey breast

Hummus

Sliced bell peppers

Sliced cucumbers

Baby spinach leaves

Preparation:

Lay out a slice of turkey breast.

Spread a layer of hummus.

Add sliced vegetables and baby spinach.

Roll up the turkey to create a roll-up.

8. Brain-Boosting Trail Mix

Ingredients:

Mixed nuts (e.g., almonds, walnuts, cashews)

Dried cranberries

Dark chocolate chips

Air-popped popcorn

Preparation:

Combine mixed nuts, dried cranberries, dark chocolate chips, and air-popped popcorn in a bowl.

Mix well.

Portion into small bags for on-the-go snacks.

9. Brainy Veggie Dip

Ingredients:

Baby carrots

Sliced cucumbers

Cherry tomatoes

Hummus

Preparation:

Arrange baby carrots, sliced cucumbers, and cherry tomatoes on a plate.

Serve with a side of hummus for dipping.

10. Brain-Boosting Fruit Salad

Ingredients:

Assorted fresh fruits (e.g., apples, grapes, berries, oranges)

Chopped walnuts

Greek yogurt

Honey

Preparation:

Wash and chop the fruits into bite-sized pieces.

In a bowl, mix Greek yogurt with a drizzle of honey.

Add the chopped walnuts to the yogurt and honey mixture.

Gently fold the chopped fruits into the yogurt and nut mixture

11. Brain-Boosting Berry Pancakes

Ingredients:

Whole-grain pancake mix

Mixed berries (strawberries, blueberries, raspberries)

Greek yogurt

Honey

Preparation:

Follow the directions on the package to prepare the pancake batter. Stir in mixed berries.

Cook pancakes on a griddle.

Drizzle some honey and a dollop of Greek yogurt on top.

12. Smarty Smoothie Bowl

Ingredients:

Blended smoothie (use your favorite recipe)

Sliced bananas

Chia seeds

Sliced almonds

Shredded coconut

Preparation:

Prepare a smoothie of your choice and pour it into a bowl.

Top with sliced bananas, chia seeds, sliced almonds, and shredded coconut for added brain-boosting goodness.

13. Brainy Baked Sweet Potato Fries

Ingredients:

Sweet potatoes, peeled and sliced into fries

Olive oil

Paprika

Garlic powder

Salt and pepper

Preparation:

Preheat the oven to 425°F (220°C).

Add olive oil, paprika, garlic powder, salt, and pepper to sweet potato fries.

Spread them on a baking sheet.

Bake for 25-30 minutes, turning once until they are golden and crispy.

14. Smarty Tuna Salad

Ingredients:

Canned tuna, drained

Greek yogurt

Diced celery

Diced red onion

Dill pickle relish

Mustard

Salt and pepper

Preparation: In a bowl, mix canned tuna, Greek yogurt, diced celery, diced red onion, dill pickle relish, mustard, salt, and pepper.Serve as a sandwich, wrap, or over a bed of greens.

Ingredients:

Whole-grain pita pockets

Hummus

Sliced cucumber

Sliced cherry tomatoes

Sliced bell peppers

Baby spinach leaves

Preparation:

Cut a pita pocket in half to create two pockets.

Spread hummus inside each pocket.

Fill with sliced cucumber, cherry tomatoes, bell peppers, and baby spinach.

Ingredients:

Fresh broccoli florets

Olive oil

Parmesan cheese

Garlic powder

Salt and pepper

Preparation:

Preheat the oven to 425°F (220°C).

Toss broccoli florets with olive oil, grated Parmesan cheese, garlic powder, salt, and pepper.

Spread them on a baking sheet.

Roast for 20-25 minutes until they are tender and slightly crispy.

17. Smarty Spinach and Feta Quesadilla

Ingredients:

Whole-wheat tortilla

Sliced spinach

Crumbled feta cheese

Sliced black olives

Preparation:

Place a tortilla in a heated skillet.

Sprinkle with sliced spinach, crumbled feta cheese, and sliced black olives.

Top with another tortilla.

Cook until tortillas are golden brown and cheese is melted.

18. Brain-Boosting Oatmeal Cookies

Ingredients:

Rolled oats

Whole-wheat flour

Baking powder

Ground flaxseed

Cinnamon

Mashed bananas

Unsweetened applesauce

Raisins

Preparation:

In a bowl, combine rolled oats, whole-wheat flour, baking powder, ground flaxseed, and cinnamon.

In another bowl, mix mashed bananas, unsweetened applesauce, and raisins.

Combine wet and dry ingredients.

Drop spoonful's onto a baking sheet and bake at 350°F (175°C) for 10-12 minutes.

19. Smarty Nut Butter and Banana Sushi

Ingredients:

Whole-wheat tortilla

Nut butter (peanut or almond)
Banana

Honey

Preparation:

Lay out a whole-wheat tortilla.

Spread nut butter on it.

Place a banana on one end and drizzle with honey.

Roll up the tortilla and slice into sushi-like pieces.

20. Brainy Trail Mix Energy Bites

Ingredients:

Rolled oats

Chopped nuts (e.g., almonds, walnuts)

Dried cranberries

Dark chocolate chips

Honey

Preparation:

In a bowl, mix rolled oats, chopped nuts, dried cranberries, dark chocolate chips, and honey.

Roll into bite-sized energy bites and refrigerate.

21. Brainy Berry Oat Bars

Ingredients:

Rolled oats
Mixed berries (strawberries, blueberries, raspberries)

Greek yogurt

Honey

Preparation:

In a bowl, mix rolled oats, Greek yogurt, and honey.

In a baking dish, press half of the mixture into the bottom.

Layer mixed berries on top.

Add the remaining oat mixture over the berries.

Refrigerate for a few hours, then cut into bars.

22. Smarty Pita Pizza

Ingredients:

Whole-grain pita bread

Tomato sauce

Sliced bell peppers

Sliced cherry tomatoes

Sliced black olives

Shredded mozzarella cheese

Preparation:

Preheat the oven to 375°F (190°C).

Place a whole-grain pita on a baking sheet.

Spread tomato sauce and add sliced vegetables.

Top with shredded mozzarella cheese.

Bake for 10-12 minutes or until cheese is bubbly and slightly golden.

23. Brain-Boosting Turkey Meatballs

Ingredients:

Ground turkey

Rolled oats

Grated zucchini

Diced onions

Garlic powder

Salt and pepper

Preparation:

In a bowl, mix ground turkey, rolled oats, grated zucchini, diced onions, garlic powder, salt, and pepper.

Form into meatballs and bake at 375°F (190°C) for 20-25 minutes.

24. Smarty Cheesy Quesadilla

Ingredients:

Whole-wheat tortilla

Shredded cheddar cheese

Sliced avocado

Sliced cherry tomatoes

Sliced black olives

Preparation:

Place a whole-wheat tortilla in a heated skillet.

Sprinkle with shredded cheddar cheese.

Add sliced avocado, cherry tomatoes, and black olives.

Top with another tortilla.

Cook until cheese is melted and tortillas are golden brown.

25. Brainy Banana Blueberry Muffins

Ingredients:

Whole-wheat flour

Baking powder

Baking soda

Ground flaxseed

Mashed bananas

Blueberries

Greek yogurt

Honey

Preparation:

In a bowl, combine whole-wheat flour, baking powder, baking soda, and ground flaxseed.

Stir in mashed bananas, blueberries, Greek yogurt, and honey.

Pour into muffin cups and bake at 350°F (175°C) for 15-20 minutes.

26. Brain-Boosting Cucumber Boats

Ingredients:

Cucumber

Tuna salad (as in recipe #14)

Cherry tomatoes

Preparation:

Cut a cucumber in half lengthwise and scoop out the seeds to create a "boat."

Fill the cucumber boat with tuna salad.

Garnish with cherry tomato halves.

27. Brainy Spinach and Feta Omelet

Ingredients:

Eggs

Chopped spinach

Crumbled feta cheese

Salt and pepper

Preparation:

Whisk eggs in a bowl and season with salt and pepper.

Pour the eggs into a heated skillet.

Add chopped spinach and crumbled feta cheese.

Cook until the eggs are set, then fold in half.

28. Smarty Celery and Peanut Butter Logs

Ingredients:

Celery sticks

Peanut butter (or almond butter)

Raisins

Preparation:

Fill celery sticks with peanut butter.

Top with raisins for added flavor and nutrition.

29. Brain-Boosting Fruit and Nut Parfait

Ingredients:

Greek yogurt

Chopped mixed nuts (e.g., almonds, walnuts)

Diced fresh fruits (e.g., apples, berries, oranges)

Honey

Preparation:

In a glass or jar, layer Greek yogurt, mixed nuts, and diced fresh fruits.

Drizzle with honey for added sweetness.

30. Brainy Avocado and Egg Toast

Ingredients:

Whole-grain bread

Avocado slices

Poached or fried egg

Sliced tomatoes

Sliced radishes

Sprouts (e.g., alfalfa)

Preparation:

Toast whole-grain bread.

Spread avocado slices on the toast.

Top with a poached or fried egg.

Garnish with sliced tomatoes, radishes, and sprouts.

31. Smarty Spinach and Cheese Quesadilla

Ingredients:

Whole-wheat tortilla

Sliced spinach

Shredded cheddar cheese

Sliced mushrooms

Sliced bell peppers

Preparation:

Place a whole-wheat tortilla in a heated skillet.

Sprinkle with shredded cheddar cheese.

Add sliced spinach, mushrooms, and bell peppers.

Top with another tortilla.

Cook the tortillas until they are golden brown and the cheese has melted.

32. Brainy Banana Walnut Muffins

Ingredients:

Whole-wheat flour

Baking powder

Ground flaxseed

Mashed bananas

Chopped walnuts

Greek yogurt

Honey

Preparation:

In a bowl, combine whole-wheat flour, baking powder, and ground flaxseed.

Stir in mashed bananas, chopped walnuts, Greek yogurt, and honey.

Pour into muffin cups and bake at 350°F (175°C) for 15-20 minutes.

33. Brain-Boosting Chicken and Veggie Nuggets

Ingredients:

Ground chicken

chopped mixed vegetables, such as bell peppers, broccoli, and carrots

Breadcrumbs

Egg

Garlic powder

Salt and pepper

Preparation:

In a bowl, combine ground chicken, chopped mixed vegetables, breadcrumbs, egg, garlic powder, salt, and pepper.

Shape into nuggets and bake at 375°F (190°C) for 20-25 minutes.

34. Smarty Apple and Cheese Quesadilla

Ingredients:

Whole-wheat tortilla

Sliced apples

Shredded cheddar cheese

Cinnamon

Preparation:

Place a whole-wheat tortilla in a heated skillet.

Sprinkle with shredded cheddar cheese.

Add some apple slices and a pinch of cinnamon.

Top with another tortilla.

Cook the tortillas until they are golden brown and the cheese has melted.

35. Brainy Broccoli and Cheese Stuffed Potatoes

Ingredients:

Baked potatoes

Broccoli florets

Shredded cheddar cheese

Greek yogurt

Salt and pepper

Preparation:

Cut open baked potatoes.

Fill with steamed broccoli florets, shredded cheddar cheese, Greek yogurt, salt, and pepper.

Place under a broiler for a few minutes until cheese is bubbly.

36. Brainy Almond and Date Energy Bites

Ingredients:

Almonds

Dates

Rolled oats

Cinnamon

Preparation:

In a food processor, blend almonds, dates, rolled oats, and a dash of cinnamon until the mixture sticks together.

Roll into bite-sized energy bites and refrigerate.

37. Smarty Turkey and Cheese Wrap

Ingredients:

Whole-grain wrap

Sliced turkey

Sliced cheddar cheese

Sliced apples

Lettuce

Preparation:

Lay out a whole-grain wrap.

Layer sliced turkey, cheddar cheese, sliced apples, and lettuce.

Roll up and slice into bite-sized pieces.

Ingredients:

Whole-wheat flour

Baking powder

Ground flaxseed

Shredded carrots

Raisins

Greek yogurt

Honey

Preparation:

In a bowl, combine whole-wheat flour, baking powder, and ground flaxseed.

Stir in shredded carrots, raisins, Greek yogurt, and honey.

Pour into muffin cups and bake at 350°F (175°C) for 15-20 minutes.

Ingredients:

Eggs

Chopped mixed vegetables (e.g., broccoli, bell peppers, spinach)

Shredded cheddar cheese
Salt and pepper

Preparation:

Whisk eggs in a bowl and season with salt and pepper.

In a muffin tin, distribute chopped mixed vegetables and shredded cheddar cheese.

Over the veggies and cheese, pour the egg mixture.

Bake at 350°F (175°C) for 15-20 minutes.

40. Brainy Sweet Potato Fries

Ingredients:

Sweet potatoes

Olive oil

Paprika

Salt and pepper

Preparation:

Cut sweet potatoes into fries.

Add salt, pepper, paprika, and olive oil and toss.

Bake at 400°F (200°C) for 20-25 minutes or until crispy.

41. Brainy Lentil and Vegetable Soup

Ingredients:

Green or brown lentils

Chopped mixed vegetables (e.g., carrots, celery, onions)
Low-sodium vegetable broth

Spices (e.g., cumin, paprika, thyme)

Preparation:

In a pot, sauté chopped mixed vegetables until tender.

Add lentils, spices, and low-sodium vegetable broth.

Simmer until lentils are cooked through and vegetables are soft.

42. Smarty Pineapple and Cheese Quesadilla

Ingredients:

Whole-wheat tortilla

Sliced pineapple

Shredded mozzarella cheese

Sliced ham (optional)

Preparation:

Place a whole-wheat tortilla in a heated skillet.

Sprinkle with shredded mozzarella cheese.

Add sliced pineapple and, if desired, sliced ham.

Top with another tortilla.

Cook the tortillas until they are golden brown and the cheese has melted.

43. Brainy Banana Peanut Butter Smoothie

Ingredients:

Banana

Peanut butter (or almond butter)

Greek yogurt

Honey

Milk (dairy or plant-based)

Preparation:

Blend banana, peanut butter, Greek yogurt, honey, and milk until smooth.

44. Smarty Turkey and Veggie Wrap

Ingredients:

Whole-grain wrap

Sliced turkey

Sliced cheddar cheese

Sliced cucumbers

Sliced bell peppers

Lettuce

Preparation:

Lay out a whole-grain wrap.

Layer sliced turkey, cheddar cheese, cucumbers, bell peppers, and lettuce.

Roll up and slice into bite-sized pieces.

45. Brain-Boosting Chocolate Avocado Pudding

Ingredients:

Ripe avocados

Cocoa powder

Honey

Vanilla extract

Milk (dairy or plant-based)

Preparation:

Blend ripe avocados, cocoa powder, honey, vanilla extract, and a splash of milk until smooth.

Chill in the refrigerator before serving.

46. Brainy Tofu and Veggie Stir-Fry

Ingredients:

Tofu

Chopped mixed vegetables (e.g., broccoli, bell peppers, snap peas)

Low-sodium stir-fry sauce

Brown rice

Preparation:

Cube tofu and sauté until golden brown.

Add chopped mixed vegetables and low-sodium stir-fry sauce.

Serve over cooked brown rice.

47. Smarty Almond Butter and Banana Wrap

Ingredients:

Whole-grain wrap

Almond butter

Banana

Honey

Preparation:

Lay out a whole-grain wrap.

Spread almond butter on it.

Place a banana and drizzle with honey.

Roll up and slice into bite-sized pieces.

48. Brainy Chickpea Salad

Ingredients:

Chickpeas (canned or cooked)

Chopped cucumbers

Chopped tomatoes

Chopped red onions

Feta cheese

Olive oil and balsamic vinegar

Preparation:

In a bowl, combine chickpeas, cucumbers, tomatoes, red onions, and feta cheese.

Drizzle with olive oil and balsamic vinegar.

49. Smarty Veggie and Hummus Wrap

Ingredients:

Whole-grain wrap

Hummus

Sliced cucumbers

Sliced bell peppers

Sliced cherry tomatoes

Sliced black olives

Preparation:

Lay out a whole-grain wrap.

Spread hummus on it.

Layer sliced cucumbers, bell peppers, cherry tomatoes, and black olives.

Roll up and slice into bite-sized pieces.

50. Brain-Boosting Berry and Spinach Smoothie

Ingredients:

Baby spinach

Mixed berries (e.g., blueberries, strawberries, raspberries)

Greek yogurt

Honey

Milk (dairy or plant-based)

Preparation:

Blend baby spinach, mixed berries, Greek yogurt, honey, and milk until smooth.

51.Smarty Blueberry and Banana Pancakes

Ingredients:

Whole-wheat flour

Baking powder

Mashed bananas

Blueberries

Milk (dairy or plant-based)

Preparation:

In a bowl, mix whole-wheat flour, baking powder, mashed bananas, blueberries, and milk.

On a griddle, cook pancakes until golden brown.

52. Brainy Quinoa and Black Bean Salad

Ingredients:

Cooked quinoa

Black beans

Corn kernels

Diced tomatoes

Avocado

Cilantro

Lime juice

Preparation:

Combine cooked quinoa, black beans, corn kernels, diced tomatoes, and avocado.

Add cilantro as a garnish and squeeze lime juice over it.

53. Smarty Turkey and Veggie Meatballs

Ingredients:

Ground turkey

Chopped mixed vegetables (e.g., carrots, bell peppers)

Breadcrumbs

Egg

Garlic powder

Salt and pepper

Preparation:

In a bowl, mix ground turkey, chopped mixed vegetables, breadcrumbs, egg, garlic powder, salt, and pepper.

Form into meatballs, then place in the oven to bake.

54. Brain-Boosting Green Bean Fries

Ingredients:

Fresh green beans

Whole-wheat breadcrumbs

Parmesan cheese

Olive oil

Garlic powder

Preparation:

Toss green beans in olive oil, garlic powder, and breadcrumbs with grated Parmesan cheese.

Bake until crispy.

55. Smarty Pita Bread Pizza

Ingredients:

Whole-grain pita bread

Tomato sauce

Shredded mozzarella cheese

Sliced vegetables (e.g., bell peppers, cherry tomatoes)

Preparation:

Spread tomato sauce on whole-grain pita bread.

Sprinkle with shredded mozzarella cheese and add sliced vegetables.

Bake until cheese is melted.

56. Brainy Veggie and Cheese Omelette

Ingredients:

Eggs

Chopped mixed vegetables (e.g., spinach, bell peppers, onions)

Shredded cheddar cheese

Olive oil

Salt and pepper

Preparation:

In a bowl, whisk together eggs and add pepper and salt to taste.

Sauté chopped mixed vegetables in olive oil until tender.

Pour the egg mixture over the vegetables and sprinkle with shredded cheddar cheese.

Cook until set and fold in half.

57. Smarty Cucumber and Cream Cheese Sandwiches

Ingredients:

Whole-grain bread

Cream cheese

Sliced cucumbers

Dill (optional)

Preparation:

Spread cream cheese on whole-grain bread.

Layer with sliced cucumbers and dill, if desired.

58. Brainy Coconut and Berry Parfait

Ingredients:

Greek yogurt

Mixed berries (e.g., strawberries, blueberries)

Shredded coconut

Honey

Preparation:

Layer Greek yogurt with mixed berries, shredded coconut, and drizzles of honey in a glass or bowl.

59. Smarty Sweet Potato and Cinnamon Muffins

Ingredients:

Sweet potatoes

Whole-wheat flour

Baking powder
Cinnamon

Greek yogurt

Honey

Preparation:

Cook and mash sweet potatoes.

In a bowl, combine mashed sweet potatoes, whole-wheat flour, baking powder, cinnamon, Greek yogurt, and honey.

Pour into muffin cups and bake until golden brown.

60. Brainy Salmon and Veggie Foil Packets

Ingredients:

Salmon fillets

Sliced mixed vegetables (e.g., zucchini, bell peppers, carrots)

Lemon slices

Olive oil

Herbs (e.g., dill, parsley)

Preparation:

Place salmon fillets on a piece of aluminum foil.

Top with sliced mixed vegetables, lemon slices, a drizzle of olive oil, and herbs.

Seal the foil into packets and bake until the salmon flakes easily.

61. Smarty Veggie and Cheese Quesadillas

Ingredients:

Whole-wheat tortillas

Sliced bell peppers

Sliced zucchini

Preparation:

Place a whole-wheat tortilla in a heated skillet.

Sprinkle with shredded cheese and add sliced bell peppers and zucchini.

Top with another tortilla.

Cook until the tortillas are golden brown and the cheese has melted.

62. Brain-Boosting Carrot and Raisin Salad

Ingredients:

Grated carrots

Raisins

Greek yogurt

Honey

Lemon juice

Preparation:

In a bowl, combine grated carrots and raisins.

In a separate bowl, mix Greek yogurt, honey, and lemon juice.

Drizzle the yogurt mixture over the carrot and raisin salad.

63. Smarty Apple and Cheese Wraps

Ingredients:

Whole-grain wrap

Sliced apples

Sliced cheddar cheese

Honey (optional)

Preparation:

Lay out a whole-grain wrap.

Layer sliced apples and cheddar cheese.

Drizzle with honey, if desired.

Roll up and slice into bite-sized pieces.

64. Brainy Turkey and Vegetable Stir-Fry

Ingredients:

Ground turkey

Mixed vegetables (e.g., broccoli, carrots, snow peas)

Low-sodium stir-fry sauce

Brown rice

Preparation:

Cook the ground turkey in a skillet until browned. Add mixed vegetables and stir-fry sauce.

Serve over cooked brown rice.

65. Smarty Banana and Almond Butter Roll-Ups

Ingredients:

Whole-grain tortillas

Almond butter

Sliced bananas

Preparation:

Spread almond butter on a whole-grain tortilla.

Add sliced bananas.

Roll up and slice into bite-sized pieces.

66. Brainy Spinach and Cheese Stuffed Mushrooms

Ingredients:

Baby spinach

Cream cheese

Parmesan cheese

Garlic powder

Mushrooms

Preparation:

Sauté baby spinach until wilted.

Mix cream cheese, Parmesan cheese, and garlic powder with the spinach.

Stuff mushroom caps with the mixture and bake until bubbly.

67. Smarty Honey and Fruit Yogurt Parfait

Ingredients:

Greek yogurt

Sliced strawberries

Blueberries

Honey

Preparation:

Layer Greek yogurt with sliced strawberries and blueberries in a glass.

Drizzle with honey.

68. Brainy Tuna Salad Lettuce Wraps

Ingredients:

Canned tuna

Greek yogurt

Chopped celery

Chopped red onion

Lettuce leaves

Preparation:

In a bowl, combine canned tuna, Greek yogurt, chopped celery, and chopped red onion.

Spoon the mixture into lettuce leaves and roll them up.

69. Smarty Cherry Tomatoes and Mozzarella Skewers

Ingredients:

Cherry tomatoes

Fresh mozzarella balls

Basil leaves

Balsamic glaze

Preparation:

Cherry tomatoes, freshly made mozzarella balls, and basil leaves should be twisted onto skewers.

Drizzle with balsamic glaze.

70. Brainy Pumpkin and Oatmeal Muffins

Ingredients:

Canned pumpkin

Rolled oats

Eggs

Cinnamon

Nutmeg

Maple syrup

Preparation:

Mix canned pumpkin, rolled oats, eggs, cinnamon, nutmeg, and maple syrup in a bowl.

Pour into muffin cups and bake until firm.

71. Smarty Turkey and Veggie Quesadillas

Ingredients:

Whole-wheat tortillas

Ground turkey

Sliced bell peppers

Sliced onions

Shredded cheddar cheese

Preparation:

Cook the ground turkey in a skillet until browned. Place a whole-wheat tortilla in a heated skillet.

Sprinkle with shredded cheddar cheese, add the cooked turkey, sliced bell peppers, and onions.

Top with another tortilla.

Cook until the tortillas are golden brown and the cheese has melted.

Ingredients:

Whole-grain bread

Avocado

Sliced tomatoes

Salt and pepper

Preparation:

Toast slices of whole-grain bread.

Spread mashed avocado on the toast and top with sliced tomatoes.

Season with salt and pepper.

73. Smarty Chickpea and Veggie Stir-Fry

Ingredients:

Cooked chickpeas

Mixed vegetables (e.g., broccoli, carrots, snap peas)

Low-sodium stir-fry sauce

Quinoa

Preparation:

Sauté cooked chickpeas and mixed vegetables in a pan with low-sodium stir-fry sauce.

Serve over cooked quinoa.

Ingredients:

Strawberries

Banana

Greek yogurt

Milk (dairy or plant-based)

Honey

Preparation:

Blend strawberries, banana, Greek yogurt, milk, and honey until smooth.

Ingredients:

Whole-grain wrap

Sliced turkey

Cranberry sauce

Sliced cucumbers

Sliced red onion

Preparation:

Lay out a whole-grain wrap.

Layer sliced turkey, cranberry sauce, sliced cucumbers, and red onion.

Roll up and slice into bite-sized pieces.

76. Brainy Broccoli and Cheese Bites

Ingredients:

Chopped broccoli

Cheddar cheese

Breadcrumbs

Eggs

Garlic powder

Salt and pepper

Preparation:

Steam chopped broccoli until tender.

In a bowl, mix broccoli, cheddar cheese, breadcrumbs, eggs, garlic powder, salt, and pepper.

Shape into bites and bake until golden brown.

77. Smarty Raspberry and Almond Butter Sandwich

Ingredients:

Whole-grain bread

Almond butter

Raspberries

Preparation:
Spread almond butter on whole-grain bread.

Layer with raspberries.

Press another slice of bread on top.

78. Brainy Spinach and Tomato Quesadillas

Ingredients:

Whole-wheat tortillas

Baby spinach

Sliced tomatoes

Shredded mozzarella cheese

Preparation:

Place a whole-wheat tortilla in a heated skillet.

Sprinkle with shredded mozzarella cheese, add baby spinach and sliced tomatoes.

Top with another tortilla.

Cook until the tortillas are golden brown and the cheese has melted.

79. Smarty Turkey and Apple Wrap

Ingredients:

Whole-grain wrap

Sliced turkey

Sliced apples

Honey mustard

Preparation:

Lay out a whole-grain wrap.

Layer sliced turkey, sliced apples, and drizzle with honey mustard.

Roll up and slice into bite-sized pieces.

80. Brain-Boosting Mango and Banana Smoothie

Ingredients:

Mango

Banana

Greek yogurt

Milk (dairy or plant-based)

Vanilla extract

Preparation:

Blend mango, banana, Greek yogurt, milk, and vanilla extract until smooth.

81. Smarty Sweet Potato Fries

Ingredients:

Sweet potatoes

Olive oil

Paprika

Garlic powder

Salt and pepper

Preparation:

Cut sweet potatoes into fry-like shapes.

Add salt, pepper, paprika, garlic powder, and olive oil and toss.

Bake until crispy.

82. Brainy Tuna and Cucumber Rolls

Ingredients:

Canned tuna

Cucumber

Greek yogurt

Dill

Lemon juice

Preparation:

In a bowl, mix canned tuna, Greek yogurt, dill, and lemon juice.

Slice cucumber into long strips.

Spread the tuna mixture on cucumber strips and roll them up.

83. Smarty Pomegranate and Yogurt Parfait

Ingredients:

Greek yogurt

Pomegranate seeds

Granola

Honey

Preparation:

Layer Greek yogurt with pomegranate seeds, granola, and drizzles of honey in a glass or bowl.

84. Brain-Boosting Tofu and Veggie Stir-Fry

Ingredients:

Extra-firm tofu

Mixed vegetables (e.g., bell peppers, broccoli, carrots)

Low-sodium stir-fry sauce

Brown rice

Preparation:

Cube tofu and sauté until lightly browned.

Add mixed vegetables and stir-fry sauce.

Serve over cooked brown rice.

85. Smarty Apple Slices with Almond Butter

Ingredients:

Apple slices

Almond butter

Cinnamon (optional)

Preparation:

Spread almond butter on apple slices.

Sprinkle with cinnamon, if desired.

86. Brainy Turkey and Cheese Pinwheels

Ingredients:

Whole-wheat tortillas

Sliced turkey

Sliced cheddar cheese

Spinach leaves

Preparation:

Lay out a whole-wheat tortilla.

Layer sliced turkey, cheddar cheese, and spinach leaves.

Roll up and slice into bite-sized pinwheels.

87. Smarty Cherry and Almond Muffins

Ingredients:

Cherries (fresh or frozen)

Almond meal

Eggs

Honey

Almond extract

Preparation:

Mix cherries, almond meal, eggs, honey, and almond extract in a bowl.

Pour into muffin cups and bake until firm.

88. Brain-Boosting Roasted Red Pepper Hummus

Ingredients:

Canned chickpeas

Roasted red peppers

Tahini

Lemon juice

Garlic

Olive oil

Preparation:

Blend garlic, tahini, lemon juice, roasted red peppers, and chickpeas until smooth.

Drizzle with olive oil and serve with veggie sticks or whole-wheat pita.

89. Smarty Carrot and Orange Smoothie

Ingredients:

Carrots

Oranges

Greek yogurt

Honey

Preparation:

Blend carrots, oranges, Greek yogurt, and honey until smooth.

90. Brainy Quinoa and Veggie Stuffed Peppers

Ingredients:

Bell peppers

Cooked quinoa

Mixed vegetables (e.g., corn, black beans, tomatoes)

Taco seasoning

Preparation:

Remove the seeds from bell peppers by cutting off the tops.

In a bowl, mix cooked quinoa, mixed vegetables, and taco seasoning.

Stuff the bell peppers and bake until peppers are tender.

91. Smarty Berry and Spinach Salad

Ingredients:

Baby spinach

Mixed berries (e.g., strawberries, blueberries, raspberries)

Feta cheese

Balsamic vinaigrette

Preparation:

Combine baby spinach, mixed berries, and crumbled feta cheese in a bowl.

Drizzle with balsamic vinaigrette.

92. Brainy Pumpkin and Banana Muffins

Ingredients:

Canned pumpkin

Mashed bananas

Whole-wheat flour

Baking powder

Cinnamon

Nutmeg

Preparation:

Mix canned pumpkin, mashed bananas, whole-wheat flour, baking powder, cinnamon, and nutmeg in a bowl.

Fill muffin tins, then bake until golden.

93. Smarty Peanut Butter and Banana Toast

Ingredients:

Whole-grain bread

Peanut butter

Sliced bananas

Honey (optional)

Preparation:

Toast slices of whole-grain bread.

After spreading peanut butter on the toast, place sliced bananas on top.

Drizzle with honey, if desired.

94. Brain-Boosting Pita Pocket Snacks

Ingredients:

Whole-grain mini pita pockets

Hummus

Sliced cucumbers

Sliced bell peppers

Preparation:

Cut mini pita pockets in half.

Spread hummus inside and stuff with sliced cucumbers and bell peppers.

95. Smarty Blueberry and Almond Oatmeal

Ingredients:

Rolled oats

Almond milk

Blueberries

Almond slices

Preparation:

Cook rolled oats in almond milk.

Top with blueberries and almond slices.

96. Brainy Veggie and Cheese Stuffed Baked Potatoes

Ingredients:

Baked potatoes

Broccoli florets

Cheddar cheese

Greek yogurt

Chives

Preparation:

Bake potatoes until tender.

Steam broccoli florets.

Slice open the potatoes and stuff with broccoli, cheddar cheese, Greek yogurt, and chives.

97. Smarty Turkey and Veggie Omelette

Ingredients:

Eggs
Ground turkey

Chopped mixed vegetables (e.g., spinach, mushrooms, bell peppers)

Salsa

Preparation:

Whisk eggs in a bowl.

Cook the ground turkey until browned in a skillet.

Cook the chopped mixed vegetables until they become tender. Pour the whisked eggs over the mixture and cook until set.

Top with salsa.

98. Brain-Boosting Banana and Spinach Pancakes

Ingredients:

Spinach

Mashed bananas

Whole-wheat flour

Baking powder

Preparation:

Blend spinach with mashed bananas until smooth.

Mix the spinach and banana mixture with whole-wheat flour and baking powder.

Pancakes should be griddle-cooked until golden brown.

Ingredients:

Chia seeds

Almond milk

Vanilla extract

Berries (e.g., strawberries, blueberries)

Preparation:

In a jar, combine almond milk, chia seeds, and vanilla extract.

Refrigerate overnight.

Top with berries before serving.

Ingredients:

Zucchini

Whole-wheat breadcrumbs

Parmesan cheese

Olive oil

Italian seasoning

Preparation:

Cut zucchini into fry-like shapes.

Toss with whole-wheat breadcrumbs, grated Parmesan cheese, olive oil, and Italian seasoning.

Bake until crispy.

101. Smarty Apple and Carrot Slaw

Ingredients:

Apples

Carrots

Greek yogurt

Lemon juice

Honey

Preparation:

Grate apples and carrots.

In a bowl, combine grated apples, grated carrots, Greek yogurt, lemon juice, and honey.

102. Brainy Tofu and Veggie Nuggets

Ingredients:

Extra-firm tofu

Mixed vegetables (e.g., broccoli, carrots, corn)

Whole-wheat breadcrumbs

Eggs

Italian seasoning

Preparation:
Cube tofu.

Steam mixed vegetables until tender.

Dip tofu and veggies in beaten eggs, then coat with whole-wheat breadcrumbs mixed with Italian seasoning.

Bake until golden brown.

103. Smarty Cucumber and Yogurt Dip

Ingredients:

Cucumber

Greek yogurt

Garlic

Dill

Lemon juice

Preparation:

Grate cucumber.

In a bowl, mix grated cucumber, Greek yogurt, minced garlic, dill, and lemon juice.

Serve as a dip for veggie sticks.

104. Brain-Boosting Berry and Spinach Smoothie Bowl

Ingredients:

Baby spinach

Mixed berries (e.g., blueberries, raspberries)

Greek yogurt

Granola

Preparation:

Blend baby spinach, mixed berries, and Greek yogurt until smooth.

Pour into a bowl and top with granola.

105. Smarty Turkey and Veggie Tacos

Ingredients:

Ground turkey

Chopped mixed vegetables (e.g., bell peppers, onions)

Whole-grain taco shells

Salsa

Preparation:

Cook the ground turkey in a skillet until browned.

When the mixed vegetables are tender, add them chopped.

Fill whole-grain taco shells with the turkey and veggie mixture. Top with salsa.

106. Brainy Tomato and Mozzarella Salad

Ingredients:

Cherry tomatoes
Fresh mozzarella balls

Basil leaves

Balsamic glaze

Preparation:

Halve cherry tomatoes.

Put fresh mozzarella balls, cherry tomatoes, and basil leaves on skewers.

Drizzle with balsamic glaze.

107. Smarty Broccoli and Cheddar Soup

Ingredients:

Broccoli florets

Cheddar cheese

Low-sodium vegetable broth

Milk (dairy or plant-based)

Onion

Preparation:

Steam broccoli until tender.

In a pot, sauté chopped onions, then add steamed broccoli, vegetable broth, and milk.

Simmer until the ingredients are soft.

Blend until smooth and add shredded cheddar cheese.

108. Brain-Boosting Mango and Spinach Wrap

Ingredients:

Whole-grain wrap

Mango slices

Baby spinach

Greek yogurt

Preparation:

Lay out a whole-grain wrap.

Layer with mango slices, baby spinach, and a drizzle of Greek yogurt.

Roll up and slice into bite-sized pieces.

109. Smarty Raspberry and Coconut Oatmeal

Ingredients:

Rolled oats

Coconut milk

Raspberries

Shredded coconut

Preparation:

Cook rolled oats in coconut milk.

Top with raspberries and shredded coconut.

110. Brainy Spinach and Cheese Stuffed Chicken

Ingredients:

Chicken breasts

Baby spinach

Feta cheese

Garlic

Lemon juice

Preparation:

Cut a pocket into each chicken breast.

Stuff with baby spinach, feta cheese, minced garlic, and a drizzle of lemon juice.

Bake until chicken is cooked through.

111. Smarty Kiwi and Banana Smoothie

Ingredients:

Kiwi

Banana

Greek yogurt

Almond milk

Honey

Preparation:

Blend kiwi, banana, Greek yogurt, almond milk, and honey until smooth.

112. Brainy Veggie and Cheese Stuffed Pasta Shells

Ingredients:

Large pasta shells

Ricotta cheese

Chopped mixed vegetables (e.g., zucchini, bell peppers)

Marinara sauce

Preparation:

Cook pasta shells until al dente.

Mix ricotta cheese and chopped mixed vegetables.

Stuff the cooked shells with the mixture.

Serve with marinara sauce.

113. Smarty Orange and Carrot Smoothie

Ingredients:

Oranges

Carrots

Greek yogurt

Honey

Preparation:

Blend oranges, carrots, Greek yogurt, and honey until smooth.

114. Brain-Boosting Turkey and Veggie Meatballs

Ingredients:

Ground turkey

Chopped mixed vegetables (e.g., bell peppers, zucchini)

Whole-wheat breadcrumbs

Eggs

Italian seasoning

Preparation:

Mix ground turkey, chopped mixed vegetables, whole-wheat breadcrumbs, eggs, and Italian seasoning.

Form into meatballs and cook in the oven until done.

115. Smarty Strawberry and Spinach Salad with Almonds

Ingredients:

Baby spinach

Sliced strawberries

Sliced almonds

Balsamic vinaigrette

Preparation:

Combine baby spinach, sliced strawberries, and sliced almonds in a bowl.

Drizzle with balsamic vinaigrette.

116. Brainy Lentil and Veggie Soup

Ingredients:

Red lentils

Mixed vegetables (e.g., carrots, celery, onions)

Low-sodium vegetable broth

Cumin

Coriander

Preparation:

Sauté mixed vegetables in a pot.

Add red lentils, vegetable broth, cumin, and coriander.

Simmer until the lentils are soft.

117. Smarty Banana and Chocolate Smoothie

Ingredients:

Banana

Cocoa powder

Greek yogurt
Milk (dairy or plant-based)

Honey

Preparation:

Blend banana, cocoa powder, Greek yogurt, milk, and honey until smooth.

118. Brain-Boosting Avocado and Black Bean Wrap

Ingredients:

Whole-grain wrap

Mashed avocado

Black beans

Sliced tomatoes

Cilantro

Preparation:

Lay out a whole-grain wrap.

Spread mashed avocado, black beans, sliced tomatoes, and cilantro.

Roll up and slice into bite-sized pieces.

119. Smarty Mango and Cucumber Salad

Ingredients:

Mango

Cucumber

Red onion

Lime juice

Cilantro

Preparation:

Dice mango, cucumber, and red onion.

Toss with lime juice and chopped cilantro.

120. Brainy Quinoa and Veggie Stuffed Mushrooms

Ingredients:

Mushrooms

Cooked quinoa

Mixed vegetables (e.g., spinach, red bell pepper)

Parmesan cheese

Preparation:

Remove stems from mushrooms.

Mix cooked quinoa, chopped mixed vegetables, and grated Parmesan cheese.

Stuff mushroom caps and bake until tender.

CONCLUSION

As we conclude this culinary adventure, it's evident that creating an environment of food enlightenment and exploration for children is vital. By presenting wholesome and delicious recipes, we can empower parents, caregivers, and educators to make better food choices and inspire kids to enjoy them. With a newfound appreciation for the connection between the food we eat and the growth of our intellectual capacities, we can help shape a brighter future for our children.

It's our hope that "Kid-Friendly Brainy Food" serves as a valuable resource, sparking a renewed enthusiasm for preparing meals that nourish both body and mind. By making informed choices, we can celebrate the joy of eating, the joy of learning, and the joy of creating lasting memories around the family table.

So, as you venture forth into the realm of vibrant flavors and nutritional wisdom, remember that the path to a smarter and healthier generation begins with each meal, each bite, and each shared moment of discovery. Together, we can cultivate young minds and bodies, transforming mealtimes into opportunities for growth, joy, and connection. Here's to a future filled with brilliance and vitality, one mouthwatering dish at a time.

www.ingramcontent.com/pod-product-compliance
Lightning Source LLC
Chambersburg PA
CBHW080729260726
48660CB00010B/3766